# Life Without Nipples

# Life Without Nipples

Tammy Michelle

Photography by Doug Motto, 2004
Book design by Joe Swafford, 2004

Library of Congress Control Number:        2010912074
ISBN:            Hardcover              978-1-4535-5878-2
                 Softcover              978-1-4535-5877-5
                 Ebook                  978-1-4535-5879-9

This book was printed in the United States of America.

**To order additional copies of this book, contact:**
Xlibris Corporation
1-888-795-4274
www.Xlibris.com
Orders@Xlibris.com
77959

# CONTENTS

Everyone knows someone, or is someone with cancer. This book is dedicated to the lives and memories of all those who have been touched by cancer, and share the hope of finding a cure.

Special thanks go to my family, friends, doctors, nurses, health care professionals, co-workers, and spiritual supporters who were all part of my army. The fight goes on until we win the war!

# NO MORE NIPPLES AND OTHER
# RANDOM THOUGHTS
# OF BLINDNESS
# (9/21/03)

I remember when my breast surgeon was making the case for my impending mastectomy. "If you're not that emotionally attached to them and they don't function as a significant erogenous zones (to which my husband, Frank, matter-of-factly raised his hand and interjected, "They're not."), then it's a no-brainer—let's get rid of them and the fear of this cancer ever coming back and attacking you again. Besides, you will go through reconstruction surgery and have those C cups you've always wanted."

What? No more A-cup tits? What would life be like without water bras and all those assorted padded wonders!

Yes, that's when I realized that nipples are basically just primitive hoses—and anyone who's ever breastfed babies knows exactly what I mean. My "mommy mammaries" had certainly served their purpose—nursing three kids. (My last one hung on until he was two and a half years old! That's a lot of stretching—talk about *Go Go Gadget* boobs!) And the whole erogenous zone thing had pretty much been thrown out the window with the PTSD symptoms from any thought of sexual suckling serving as a memory catalyst flooding my mind with past images of bleeding, cracked nipples being vulnerable victims of multiple hickeys brought on by incessantly sucking baby lips. It just didn't fit anymore—and I don't think it really ever did.

The thought of living without nipples wasn't analogous to "if I didn't have eyes, I couldn't see." There would be advantages: I would be able to go braless after the surgery and reconstruction (and we're talking a lifetime guarantee of no sagging!) and no more unexpected "titty hard-ons"!

"The nipples can be tattooed on," my plastic surgeon told me. Okay, I'll put it on my wish list: nipples for Christmas next year! It would be like "all I want for Christmas is my two front teeth—I mean nipples!" At least I wouldn't talk funny! It would be like an optical illusion—cool! (Another random memory invades my mind here: when describing what happens during and after a mastectomy to my class of drug—and alcohol-addicted adolescents, one of my students chimed in awe, "You ain't got no nipples, Teacher Tammy? You mean it just looks like you got two knees on yo' chest!"—now there's a visual!)

Now just how was that reconstruction going to work?

"We'll pump you up every two to three weeks and try to time it with your chemo. It will be like going through puberty, watching your breasts grow!" Interesting! That should be a trip since I missed that puberty thing the first time around!

"There will be temporary expanders with metal ports that we'll use to fill the implants. We use a stud finder to find the port." I guess plastic surgeons sometimes moonlight as carpenters from time to time.

"Then we push syringes of saline, about 100 cc at a time."

Looking back, I did identify with Sigourney Weaver on a few occasions, feeling like there was a live alien growing in there. "Doctor, can you guarantee that you're not filling me up with some sort of genetic biotechnological DNA that's going to produce some sort of cloned alien? Because I'm telling you right now that I am absolutely *not* raising any more teenagers!"

Oh, and the pain—you conveniently forgot to tell me about the pain! Skin stretching is a form of ancient torture, I'm sure.

"We have to stretch the muscles and skin to make room for the permanent implants."

"You mean there's more surgery?"

"Yes, but it won't be as traumatic as the mastectomy and first phase of reconstruction. These temporary expanders just peel right out like Velcro; then we replace them with the permanent ones. You can choose from either saline or silicone."

Decisions, decisions—I'm still reeling from that Velcro imagery. And don't give me that "you'll just experience a little discomfort" bullshit. Tylenol doesn't touch this kind of pain!

Remember, I'm the one with the expanding, hard-as-rock bowling balls in my chest! Could you just please pass the Percocet?

And yes, the implants are certainly immovable, and I have no feeling in the skin. I'm constantly afraid of accidentally bumping them without knowing it. I actually have nightmares of catching them on fire, like Robin Williams's cross-dressing character in *Mrs. Doubtfire*! I really feel like an athletic chick with massive pecs that are secretly gravitating under my armpits. No more please!

"I think she's about where she wants to be," the nurse pleads my case for no more saline fills and no more pain.

(Incidentally, the pain is similar to that of my belly stretching for nine months during each pregnancy. But the difference is that all that stretching takes place in a matter of one minute during the injections, and then again in three weeks!)

"No, no, we'll go bigger. She can handle bigger."

"Has my husband been calling you?"

"They all do, sweetheart, they all do," the doctor smiles. I knew the male ego was behind this somewhere! "I believe you're about a C-cup now!" He seems proud of his work.

"Uh, could you help me sit up? I feel top heavy."

And later, the pain comes when I'm trying to sleep, and my muscles scream with every breath and movement. Discomfort, my ass! I feel like my tits are in labor!

Sometimes, my breasts feel wet, too, like I'm leaking from the inside. But I think that has something to do with temperature control. Because when it's cold outside, the expanders seem to lose heat faster and cool my skin from the inside out—at least the skin I can feel. I keep checking for leaks out of nervous habit, but without nipples, I have no barometer that can measure and "report" temperature changes!

"We can also make some nipples by pulling some skin and tying it off, similar to origami." So what is this? My breasts can become mediums for some eastern, oriental rice paper art! Could I have matching swans, please?

It's all such a new adventure, but this I know—there *is* life without nipples. Just one thing: how do I get these things out from under my arms? One thing's for sure with the laws of physics, water *does* take the path of least resistance!

# SURVIVOR
# (10/16/03)

Talk about challenges, immunities, and tribal councils, and you have an analogy for the process of breast cancer. It's amazing how a trivial reality show can parallel such gut—wrenching personal processes. Though I haven't had to sleep with any bugs and go without showering for a month (however, I have saved money on deodorant, since chemo seems to turn off my sweat glands), I have had my share of battles trying to win "immunity" until my next "tribal council" meeting with the doctors and hospitals.

"I Will Survive" draws another parallel for me, but this one aligns with divorce. I recalled the intense anxiety, lump-in-the-throat, weight loss, and confusion I felt when I heard my breast surgeon say, "The lump is suspicious—"

"Suspicious for what—?" I blurted.

"Suspicious for malignancy."

I remembered those drowning, oxygen-deprived feelings from somewhere in my past. Ah, yes, when I was going through my first divorce. How easily my mind and body reverted to that dreaded memory, when every day felt like a year. When I wasn't sure if I was making the right decision, when many days I couldn't drag myself out of bed, when the pain was just a monster I wanted to avoid. But with cancer, the monster is attached to you, and it is draining you, and you need to cut it out of your life—in order to save your life!

Women who have gone through the pain and loss of divorce are survivors, just like women who survive breast cancer, or any cancer. And any woman who's been there knows the correlation between a bad marriage and a malignant tumor!

It seems like such a curse, that by the virtue of our gender, we are at risk of experiencing these dreaded disasters. And I am one of those lucky women to have experienced them both!

Lucky because I know I am stronger; and lucky because I beat the odds of avoiding financial and psychological destruction after my divorce; and lucky because I am beating the odds of surrendering to a disease that has the potential of affecting one out of every five women—a disease that rears its ugly head every three minutes and kills a woman every thirteen minutes!

I am lucky to have been a healthy role model for my daughters who have witnessed my actions and who now truly know the risks of being traumatized by the malignancy of an unhealthy relationship and/or becoming victimized by the destructively haunting potential of a growing tumor. Ignorance is definitely *not* bliss! To know is to understand, and knowledge is power. We must educate all of our daughters.

Initially, I panicked at the thought of what I had done to Andrea and Ali. Because of our shared DNA, they were suddenly at greater risk of getting breast cancer. They now had a family history. They needed education. Education is the only antivenom for so many poisons. So I did what I do best: I started teaching and sharing. And it gives me peace to realize that I've also taught my daughters to recognize that they possess incredible strength; and that the power of that self-confidence will remind them to hold their heads high when they make that walk to their own tribal councils—to ensure beyond a shadow of a doubt that they will *not* be voted out, and that their torch will burn on! *You go, girls! I love you!*

# YOUR SHIP CANNOT COME IN UNTIL YOU HAVE A PORT (11/11/03)

Roto-Rooter has taken on a new definition for me. I've always had a "hide and seek" circulatory system. My veins can sense the presence of a needle, and they hide from any "prying prick!"

"You need a port," my nurse friend Debbie told me. And after eight unsuccessful sticks, when I went to have my baseline bone scan, I decided she was probably right and signed up to have a porta-cath inserted in my upper right arm.

Like an alien snake charmer, the vascular surgeon cut open my arm (thank goodness for Versed!) and attempted to search for my main vein in which to thread this plastic tube on a journey toward my heart. Then there's a handy little plastic chamber that sits right under my skin and feels like a small rock. And don't bump it because it sends shivers up my arm!

It's weird now because I have to have my blood pressure taken in my leg because my left arm is out of commission due to my lymph-node removal, and my right arm can't be used as long as the port is in place. And no lifting—a gallon of milk is my limit. Does this get me out of grocery shopping?

I do, however, recommend the whole port thing. You can get them in your chest, too—which is actually more common, I think. But my *huge* breasts were a problem there since the temporary implants were too close to where the port would be placed. So the arm had to do. I am anxious to get the thing out, though. Let me know when that ship comes in!

# LOVE JUICE–MY ASS!
## (11/16/03)

"Think of it as love juice—the nectar for life," the chemo nurses would say.

Yeah, right! The shit is poison, and the whole idea of injecting me with this stuff seems so archaic. "We're going to kill the cancer cells by killing *all* of your cells." With that kind of logic, no wonder it's taking so long to find a cure for cancer! It sounds a bit like George Bush's line of convincing our nation that it was necessary to destroy Iraq to find Saddam—kind of like the needle in the haystack philosophy!

"It will be like an insurance policy so your cancer won't come back," was another "chemoism" I was told. Pretty high premium to pay for that kind of insurance! And I'm supposed to trust our health-care system!

During my oncologist's presentation (which was written on the sanitary paper cover for the examining table!), I was bombarded with the statistics of how different treatments affect breast cancer, and the realization that I was becoming one of those inhuman statistics. I heard things like, "if you have surgery and no chemo, you have this survival statistic . . . if you have lymph involvement, the statistic changes to this . . . with radiation it's this . . . and with chemo those statistics go up . . . so best-case scenario is having surgery with no lymph node involvement, followed by chemo, then your chances are almost 90 percent!"

"But I want 100 percent! Why can't I have that?"

And I remember my oncologist's conspicuously obvious response, "Look out the window. See that woman down there on the street waiting for the bus. If she's over fifty and hasn't had a mammogram, her chances are only 75 percent!"

"So by having cancer, I have a higher rate of survival—is that what you're saying?"

"Yes, that's exactly what I'm saying. And we'll be following you every year for the rest of your life."

"I guess I've just been admitted to the 'Chemo Club'! Come right in, sit right down! Baby, let it all hang out! Where's my initiation? Let me at that love juice!"

Now let's talk about some of the side effects from the chemotherapy: besides the obvious hair loss, there's the eternal desert mouth, and the cumbersome and painful mouth sores, and chapped lips (so much for those intimate mouth action moments—kissing was definitely on hold!). I drank so much water while I was going through chemo. I remember waking up every hour and a half at night when the hot flashes would rouse me from a deep sleep. My tongue would literally be stuck to the bottom and roof of my mouth. And any movement meant the skin would rip away like I was licking an ice cube! I would try to suck in just enough water to lubricate my mouth—oilcan, please!

And the havoc the chemo does to your digestive system: It hurt to swallow, and my whole esophagus burned, my stomach churned, and the peristalsis that was supposed to "move" my intestines was somehow paralyzed by the trauma. I remember spending long spans of time on the toilet trying to push between episodes of boisterous flatulence (I know, way too much information)!

"You *have* to eat!" The words echoed at every checkup.

All I can say to this is "just take the Marinol!" (More to come on that mind-expanding topic later) It *is* important to eat. But what amazed me was that even though I forced tiny bites of bland mashed potatoes and oatmeal and slurped small sips of soup, smoothies, and milkshakes (note to self: stick to the cold foods; they tend to numb the pain and taste buds), I was consistently *gaining* weight! How was this possible?

Chemo definitely follows no logical diet plan.

I ate foods that were certainly *not* part of my low-cholesterol, low-fat diet that I had adhered to with the daily swallow of my Pravachol.

"We're not worried about your cholesterol. In fact, chemo tends to lower cholesterol counts." (Hmm . . . I'm thinking of a television advertisement to compete with those tacky Lipitor ads.) "Quit taking your cholesterol medicine for now, and just eat what you can."

And I did eat—things I'd avoided for years, and some I didn't even like! I craved salt, ate salty potato chips, French fries, and barbeque chips. Bacon and sausage, red meat, and spare ribs! My husband was so happy. Being the wonderful gourmet cook that he is, Frank was finally able to fix meals with no guilt about counting calories and fat grams for me.

"You had to get cancer, for me to sway you over to the dark side, honey!" Yes, those were the good times, with no worries—that's funny now, almost as funny as the night when we laughed until we cried over a TV show *SNL* that was never really that funny before. And Frank turned to me through tear-streaked eyes, cotton-mouthed cramped cheeks, lips sticking to his teeth, and said, "This is what I want you to remember about cancer, honey—laughing our asses off in the basement on Saturday night!" I have to say that trunk monkey commercial was a hoot! *Thanks, Frank! I love you!*

The psychological side effects from the chemotherapy were probably the most annoying. No one really tells you about this hush-hush subject. But I do know that antidepressant medication is commonly prescribed to chemo patients. Sometimes I thought I was going crazy! I would forget things; I couldn't remember what I was looking for or where I was going. And sometimes my vision would blur. I was definitely ADHD! I couldn't concentrate on anything for more than ten or fifteen minutes (which is probably why it took me so long to write this book!). I had all this time on my hands, and I absolutely couldn't concentrate enough to read all the books everyone gave me. Sometimes I would just hold my bald head in my hands and try to pull the skin away from my skull in an unconscious effort, I guess, to set my brain free!

As a footnote, however, the thing that got me through the whole nightmare—especially during those dark, sleepless nights—was my wonderful husband. *You are my rock, Frank!* He never stopped loving or caring. He never pitied me or felt sorry for me. He just encouraged me everyday and held my hand and my head with his strong heart. He slept by me every night and kept me steady with his consistent vision—that we were going to get through this together.

My incredible family served as my ultimate safety net. I will be forever grateful to my mom and dad and my Aunt Janet for staying with me, nursing my every need. I cherish that time. It helped so much. But besides my phenomenal family, I think of how important it was to have the support and caring and prayers of my friends. I received over one hundred fifty cards, some from people I didn't even know. It was like a circle of love, and it made me feel safe.

My nurse friend Debbie kept everything real for me. I love her for not sugar coating the facts for me. Debbie just tells it like it is. But she is such a wealth of information. I've called upon her expertise many, many times, and often at all hours of the night, over the last twenty-four years. I think I trusted her more than the other professionals, especially during my two-day hospital stay when I had the mastectomies. Debbie spent the night with me after that surgery—in fact, she's been at all my surgeries. As far as I'm concerned, Florence Nightingale has nothing on Debbie!

I know it sounds corny, but this is true: My "country" girlfriend Lisa was my chemo buddy and one of the generals in my army in my war against cancer. She would accompany my mom, my dad, my aunt, and me to every chemo session.

And she was never without the accessory of one or two of those outrageous entertainment magazines, like the *Star* and the *Globe*. She would entertain our group of chemo buddies every three weeks with crazy stories about clown babies and believe-it-or-not cures for cancer, specifically one that had been shown to a man in a dream to cure his wife with brazil nuts and rootbeer. I particularly remember the pictorial of Osama and Saddam's wedding. We laughed and at times forgot about the needles in our arms connected to those bags and syringes of Cytoxan and fluorouracil, and the "red devil" epirubicin.

We were soldiers, fighting our battles—but Lisa never let us lose sight of our faith. "I was put here on this earth to beautify the planet! God gave me the opportunity to stray from employment, so I could have the precious time to entertain," she would confirm and affirm. And her stage was the chemotherapy treatment room at the oncology office! *We love you, Lisa!* Everyone needs a "Lisa" when going through chemo!

# WHO'S WINNING?
# THE TORTOISE OR THE HAIR?
## (10/15/03)

Slow and steady wins the race. Often, time goes so slow, so tortoise-like. But the whole hair thing is a real defining moment!

"Cut your hair short," people told me, "to avoid the shock." Okay, I've never had short hair, so I agreed to a transition.

"Just don't make me look like a lesbian." I've already succumbed to wearing comfortable shoes—and after the nouveau cut, I did get hit on by two women at the smoothie bar in a local natural foods market. Okay, this is a novel thing, but when I'm bald, will I attract psychotic alien wannabes and Mr. Clean look-alikes?

My husband's Uncle Rich shared the most humorous moment, which prepared me for the onslaught of hair loss: "I was standing in line at the urinal at a Bears game," he said, "and I felt something sliding down my pants leg. I shook my leg, and to my surprise, a pile of hair fell out around my shoes! When I opened my fly, a waterfall of pubic hair came flowing out simultaneously with the urine. Suddenly, I felt stunned by the puddle of hair in the urinal, but not as flabbergasted as the guy next in line behind me!"

Yes, the pubic hair is the first thing to go—smooth as a baby's butt! And speaking of derrieres, no more dingle berries! Yep, there's no hair back there either! Thank God, I can put off those annoying brazilian bikini waxes!

The hair on the head ordeal is a trip though. I chose to shave my head to a shiny finish one week after my first chemo treatment. The whole shedding thing was aggravating enough to deal with from the dog! My hair stylist did the deed.

"Just promise you won't cry," she pleaded. "Country" Lisa and little Isabella looked on as my Kojak scalp appeared.

"Not bad, but whoa, I have a small, yet very round and shiny, almost succulent skull! Now let's try on the wigs . . ."

And there were no tears until I went for my checkbook.

"I'm not going to charge you for shaving your head."

"Good grief, Lisa (yes, another Lisa—it seems I'm surrounded by wonderful Lisas! Big hugs for all my Lisas—"Loquacious" Lisa, "Neighbor" Lisa, and "British Maid" Lisa, too), I was fine until you refused your fee. This is the one and only time I wasn't hoping for a discount!"

And then the tears began to flow. We all cried and hugged, and cried some more. I didn't realize how much I'd miss Lisa, my hairdresser for the past thirteen years. We'd developed more than a client/stylist relationship, meeting every two months for some sort of color or perm. I stopped in to see her a couple times, and miss our talks. But geez, all the money I'm saving on hair products and services—realization of the "price of beauty"! (That reminds me, I must share my feelings on how much all this cancer stuff costs! Talk about mind boggling!)

Now the armpit hair is absent as well, and I've officially retired my razor. But this hair on my arms, the random eyelash and eyebrow strands—what's up with that? And my fingernails—they've never grown so fast! I had to take a picture one night by the fire (10/14/03) after the Cubs lost to the Marlins (8-3), just to have a memory of all five nails on my left hand growing at top speed. Just what is this race all about? My body is calling all the shots!

I remember when I found out that my daughter Andrea had started to put dread locks in her hair.

"Andrea, what do you think you're doing? Are all the art students doing this at Bowling Green? You have such beautiful hair! Why do you want to ruin it?"

"Mom, chill out! It's *only hair*!" And a light bulb went off in my brain.

"You're so right, Andrea! What was I thinking? It's *only hair*," I reflected, as I rubbed my own bald head. Out of the mouths of babes come the most unexpected wisdom!

Even though being bald was probably what I most expected, what I wasn't prepared for was how much heat is lost through the head! I've become an avid wearer of various winter hats (*Thank you, Aunt Janet!*). I know all the fabrics that prevent the most heat loss! Now if I can just get past that harrowing mirror that screams holocaust victim! That's when I smile and remind myself that this is simply my G.I. Jane phase!

Incidentally, my favorite wig moment was when I was leaving the hospital after an appointment with my oncologist.

It was raining, and I was fumbling with my umbrella. Just as I triggered the mechanism to pop open the umbrella, the end of one of the wires caught the front edge of my wig. The force was so intense that my wig flew twenty feet in the air, landing in a puddle in the driveway to the hospital parking lot. Not one of the fifteen or so people waiting for rides, smoking, and talking at the entrance said one word. They all had that stunned, stopped action look on their faces. I literally had to wave my hands and stop traffic to pick up my wig, which I just shook off and plopped back on my head. I was giggling so much, I almost peed my pants!

# MARINOL MUNCHIES . . . UNDER THE INFLUENCE (8/11/03)

This is the bomb! It definitely helps the appetite. I would recommend this for all those with a tendency toward a queasy stomach. It is prescribed to cancer patients whose symptoms of nausea and decreased appetite interfere with their physical and psychological health. I guess what makes it politically incorrect is the cumulative fear that something being so detrimental to productive life could feel so good. And it's ironic that I work in drug rehab for chemically dependent adolescents!

As far as treatment for side effects from chemotherapy, Marinol is a guaranteed comprehensive formula (at least for me, it was). The anti-nausea drugs just made me pissed off and edgy and didn't really remove any worry about the impending need to hug an occasional toilet bowl! It was on the Marinol that I discovered that I had some control over the psychological effects of nausea. I could feel physical symptoms by just thinking about getting sick. It's like everytime I see or smell bologna, I feel nauseated because it was the last thing I ate when I got the stomach flu when I was nine years old! And to this day, I can't even go by the hanging packages of bologna in the grocery store without retching!

Anyway, if my mind could actually have that much control over triggering certain physical responses, then I certainly had the capability of not feeling certain things as long as my brain was in control. I could then be faced with a challenge, instead of a threat. Amid the chaos of feeling so out of control, I knew that I indeed had the capacity to control more than I thought. (Somehow it sounded better when I was on the Marinol.)

The worst part of the whole chemo thing is that psychologically you can't do what you used to do and, furthermore, what you psychologically think you need to do. It's just depressing. And like that lady said today when I went in for my first blood count (she had been one year chemo-free), "Don't rule out depression, honey—I was better on the antidepressants." It dawned on me with obvious resolution that the depression of having cancer and being attacked with poison has to be dealt with, processed, and understood.

Making sense out of the pain makes it quicker to forget it—or maybe it's just our brain's way of burying the trauma, like childbirth. (Somehow, I don't think I'll ever forget that pain of pooping out a nine-pound watermelon . . . and what a masochist—I did it three times!)

I keep hearing voices that seem so far away (no, I'm not psychotic . . . or maybe I am . . . who said that . . . oh, yeah, I took that little pill), reminding me to keep sight of the future, and take it day by day, one day at a time. But does anyone know how f—king hard that is? (It was at this point that I empathized with the anger of a recovering alcoholic.)

There's no doubt in my mind that having breast cancer made me see the direct correlation between the disease of alcoholism and the disease of breast cancer. It's some of the same tapes: "One day at time" and "You can't control the past," and the lines from the Serenity Prayer. They all reminded me of something I'd heard at work, and something I'd lived in my personal life as well. I went back to Al-Anon for some weekly meetings, and it did seem to help. I wasn't ready for the breast cancer support groups though. Somehow, I had to be sure I was going to live through this shit before I committed to a group of women with whom I would risk my personal feelings.

But, anyway, back to the Marinol—my oncologist suggested I try the Marinol because I had absolutely no appetite, and I initially lost four pounds. The powers-that-be kind of freak out when you lose any weight. In fact, they were so pleased when the chemo was over and I started taking Arimidex every day, I'd noticed a weight gain of twenty-two pounds! I guess it's a small price to pay for the next five years!

I remember talking about my prescription to my dear psychiatrist friend Kathy, "But this is pot!"

"Tammy, you've been on benzos and opiates! My God, take the Marinol! It's the least addictive!"

"Ok, I give . . . Uncle!"

So I went to fill my prescription for Marinol, a little embarrassed to hand it over to the pharmacist, when I heard, "Uh, we don't carry this here, you'll have to go somewhere else." Excuse me, you very gladly served me a multitude of Percocets, Darvocets, and OxyContins;

oxycodone, Vicodin, Xanax, Valium, and Ativan—all of which I could have become quickly addicted to—and you can't give me any Marinol? So I went to a smaller competitor. I was amused when I read the information page included with my prescription. Under side effects was "possible euphoria," and I thought, "Damn, euphoria, now there's an ominous side effect!" I was a little perturbed that the larger, more well-known pharmaceutical chain did not carry Marinol, and wondered if some conservative ideology was involved that was politically motivated by a few right-wingers who were against any kind of legal marijuana; but I never pursued that hypothesis.

Now there's a giant issue—regarding the medical use of marijuana. I've seen both sides of this spectrum, since I've worked with chemically dependent teenagers for more than two decades. And I've certainly witnessed the debilitating consequences of habitual marijuana use and how it directly correlates with the disease of chemical dependency. But I've also learned first hand that there are benefits to marijuana used for medicinal purposes. I'm not going to go into an elaborate political speech here, but it is something worth thinking about. It's sad that there is so much futile energy and money put into alleviating something that could help so many people, but oh well, that's another book!

During my first experience with Marinol, I told my daughter Ali (who was packing for college) and her friend to keep an eye on me; and if I passed out or got sick, they would have to call 911 and tell the emergency techs that I'd taken Marinol, along with all my other medications! I really didn't know what to expect and neither did they! After about thirty minutes, I didn't feel anything significant, so I said I was going upstairs to read some of the fourth Harry Potter book that I'd been trying to finish for the past three months. I remember reading and thinking this book was extraordinarily great! I was so into the book that I hardly heard my husband calling me for dinner.

"Honey, I've never seen you eat so well after a chemo treatment! You really seem hungry!" Frank was amazed as I inhaled baked chicken breasts and noodles. Ali and Shannon started rolling their eyes and cracking up!

"Mom's got the munchies," Ali giggled. Thank God! I finally had my appetite back!

All in all, my brain and body were inundated with a variety of mind-altering substances to kill pain and make my life more manageable. At times, even the chemotherapy seemed to induce surreal and even nightmarish images that are often described during a bad acid trip. But what I tried to commit to memory were the funny things people told me that I said, and the comical moments that made me chuckle.

And so, here are some random memories from those altered states:

"Wow, you mean with this little magic button, I can just give myself morphine not just when I need it, but anytime I want it? Does that make me an addict?"—in recovery after the mastectomies.

"Have you ever seen your mom this high?"—ditto above.

"Onward, Christian soldiers going off to war . . . that reminds me of 'Zaccheus was a wee little man and a wee little man was he! He climbed up in a sycamore tree to see what he could see . . .' Lisa, find out the words to that song by the time I'm out of surgery!"—effects of Versed going off to the operating room.

"Toxic waste drugs! I really feel most guilty about the dog getting tainted by the chemo from drinking out of the toilet bowl. Frank Zappa warned us not to eat any yellow snow . . . so Rico, listen good, and don't drink any orange pee from your favorite punch bowl!"—Ativan and chemo talk.

"Could you massage my feet some more? It's the closest I can get to an orgasm right now . . . ."—post-mastectomy request.

"Thank God we all have a library of memories to choose from to form our identities. Being born to touch and be touched, to feel, to trust. Remembering the fun times makes me feel the whole truth to being alive; pain just makes you realize the power that you have. It's only natural that one would feel stronger and take more energy than the other. Sometimes it hurts to feel good, or is it good to feel hurt? I think any kind of feeling is a beautiful thing."—working through the pain.

"That was a nice talk with Andrea—I don't know if I would call it a 'Kodak moment,' but I did always wonder what it would be like to party with my kids—like taking your twenty-one-year-old out for their *first* alcoholic beverage. Some sort of rite of passage, I guess . . . like when your kids finally figure out that you're only human. What a relief to admit your vulnerabilities. I didn't realize how much of a responsibility being a parent is, and how maintaining the perfect role-model image becomes so cumulatively draining over the years. It's so important not to be seen as a hypocrite in your children's eyes. Laughing with my kids builds the memories that make me feel most alive—and assure you that your life has purpose. I feel like I've been a good parent over the years. Then my adult daughter says, 'Are you high, Mom?' I have cramps in my cheeks from smiling so much! Just call me Marinol Mom!"—under the effects of Marinol.

"What do you mean you misplaced the comforter for the bed? I mean, it's not like some pocket change or money or car keys . . . a comforter should be kind of hard to miss, hon. It *is* a rather large item. I'm sure it will turn up!"—losing my mind to chemo-brain!

"That can't be right, I must be hearing you wrong. Could you repeat that? What did you say was the name of that karaoke machine?"—discussing Christmas gifts . . . you had to be there.

# LETTER FROM THE HEART
# (9/4/03)

Communication was continually a challenge while I was going through cancer treatment. I got tired of saying the same thing over and over. "Loquacious" Lisa, Patty, and Karen relieved me from much of that redundancy. They have been my voice, and I thank them for sharing my progress with many of the people in my life. Conversely, I think it was hard for people to communicate with me as well. They didn't know what to say; and I imagine fear was a significant factor, since I'm sure many people were afraid that I was dying. Facing mortality, whether it's yours or someone else's, is never pretty.

Writing often became my therapy, as well as my method for communication. This was a letter I wrote to Frank, my dear husband, who has been there supporting me through this whole ordeal. So much of the time I found it hard to talk to anyone at all; and so this time, I decided to write a letter:

September 4, 2003

Dear Frank,

I'm not sure how I feel, I just know that I do. And sometimes I think letting out all these confusing feelings will just be a burden. But you are my best friend, and the one who I share the most with. Remember these are just my feelings, not right or wrong. And they're simply my perceptions, which at times seem to be tainted and altered by what I'm going through . . .

It's a weird feeling sometimes to watch life go on around me, almost like I'm an outsider looking in through a window.

Sometimes I feel forgotten and broken, unable to engage and enjoy what everyone else is doing. Most of the time, I just try to seem "normal" and hide how I really feel because it is just too damn scary to admit that I feel so inadequate. It's like I'm a pitiful, cancer-ridden, freak—and no one wants to hang around cancer—it might be contagious! And I think some people forget I even have cancer because I hate admitting and/or showing how debilitating it really is. I don't want people to feel sorry for me, but at the same time, I do feel better when those around me make sacrifices for me without me even asking. It is really hard for me to ask for help—and I need to learn how to do that without feeling so guilty. I've always been the one who does the helping instead of the one who desperately needs it.

It's a full-time job convincing my family and friends that I'm doing okay. But you know something? I'm *not* okay! I need you now more than ever. When I feel "good" and "almost normal," I so desperately want to share those precious moments with you. And I feel angry when life's constraints and expectations don't allow us to be together. And when I'm feeling bad and depressed, I need you then, too. You don't know how much it helps to feel you touch my hand or rub by back or just reassure me that I'm still beautiful in your eyes.

Because every time I look in the mirror or get in the shower, I see cancer. And everytime I feel pain and exhaustion, I feel cancer. And I hate it! It's like being trapped in a room with no windows or doors, feeling so alone and scared. It's like I'm being stalked and violated all the time.

I don't know if any of this makes sense to you. I don't even know if it makes sense to me sometimes. But I do know that often I get sad because you don't seem to take time to "stop and smell the roses." And I really need you to "stop and smell the roses" *with me.* I don't want time to run out—it's just too precious.

I love you,
Tammy

If I've learned anything at all, it is that *time* is our most precious commodity.

# THE LITTLE THINGS
# (4/20/04)

My son Alex turned thirteen during my cancer ordeal. The fall of his eighth-grade year, he was required to do a speech for language arts class. Assuming he would choose one of his many interests, I asked him what his topic was going to be.

"Oh, I'm doing it on breast cancer," he said.

"Why did you choose that?" I was stunned.

"Because of you, Mom," he stated so matter-of-factly.

Then I cried. I was so touched. This was a kid who never talked about anything, let alone, breast cancer. I had talked to him about my surgery of course, gave him information, encouraged him to ask questions; but he always seemed content and preoccupied with his schoolwork and sports. As he did his research for his presentation, he started realizing the scary facts about breast cancer.

"Did you know, Mom, that men can get breast cancer, too? And did you know that a woman dies every thirteen minutes from breast cancer?" The knowledge started pouring out. Alex made an awesome poster explaining the types, risk factors, and treatments for breast cancer. His teacher told me that his speech was very poignant, that when Alex started with "I did my speech on breast cancer because my mom has it . . ." all eyes and ears were on him. She said you could've heard a pin drop.

I guess it was then that I realized my cancer was indeed affecting Alex. With unconscious parental protection, I had wanted to shelter him from any trauma. Instead, what I needed to do was include him in all of what I was going through. I never talked with Alex about the risk of death from having cancer. We never talked about the fact that I could die from this disease. I tried not to even think about it. Death was just *not* an option! But that risk is there, along with so many others that can complicate our lives. It was at this time that I realized the irony of how mortality makes every piece of life seem so incredibly significant. Mortality isn't an end to life as much as it is a magnifying glass for the little things that we need to see in our lives. And I think Alex knew it, too.

Sometimes, we didn't even need to talk. He would come in from school and lie down next to me while I was sleeping off the effects of chemo. I'd wake up, and he'd be napping beside me, like a little angel. Other times I would peek my head in his room and ask him if he needed help with his homework.

"No, but you can lie down on my bed and watch me do my homework if you want to, Mom." I think it gave him comfort to have me near him. And he would tease me about my hair, and we would laugh about things that happened that day, and sometimes I'd fall asleep. I know he watched me carefully, and he started thinking hypothetically that year, experiencing abstract cognitive growth—my little boy was growing up.

I guess we've all grown up. Cancer does that to people. And it's ironic how the ordeal of removing a malignancy in an effort to cure somehow facilitates a different kind of growth, forcing you to think about what's really important. It's the little things that pile up on top of each other that form the glue that helps us accumulate all the pieces, that keeps us growing and loving and living—minute to minute, day to day, year to year. *So pile it on and raise it high, and grow, grow, grow for it—for life! There is life without nipples! I'm living proof!*

# A PICTURE'S
# WORTH A THOUSAND WORDS

I'd like to add just a footnote about the pictures. Credit needs to be given to photographer Doug Motto for organizing a photo shoot to show what cancer looks like. My objective was to share a graphic image of "Life Without Nipples."

Personally, I got so tired of seeing diagrams and cartoon pictures of mastectomy incisions and scars. I wanted to see real people with faces, so I could study their expressions and be able to understand what was going to happen to my body.

So these pictures of a real person who has had a double mastectomy and first phase of reconstruction with temporary expanders and who is going through chemotherapy. I'm the raw deal! No touchups or airbrushing, just skin, scars, and emotion! I am a *survivor*!

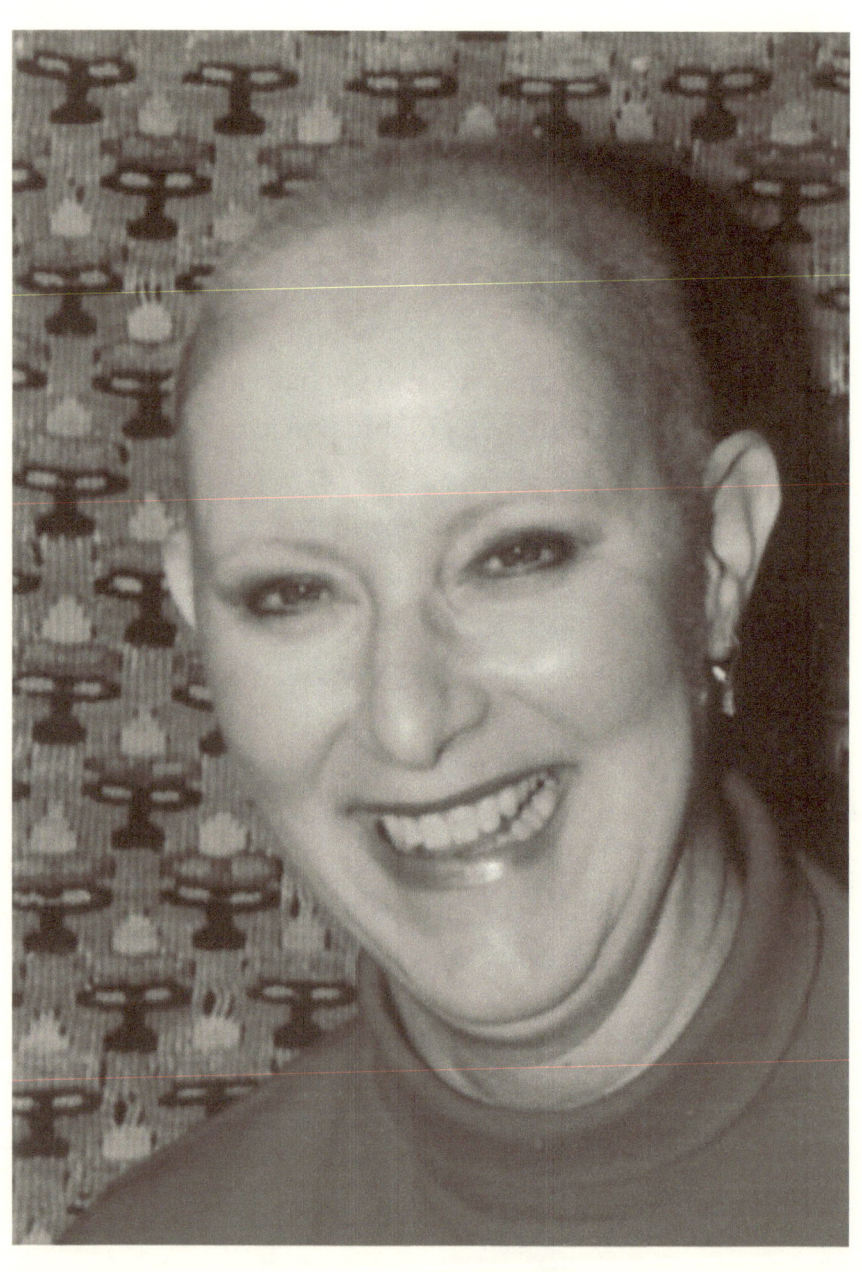

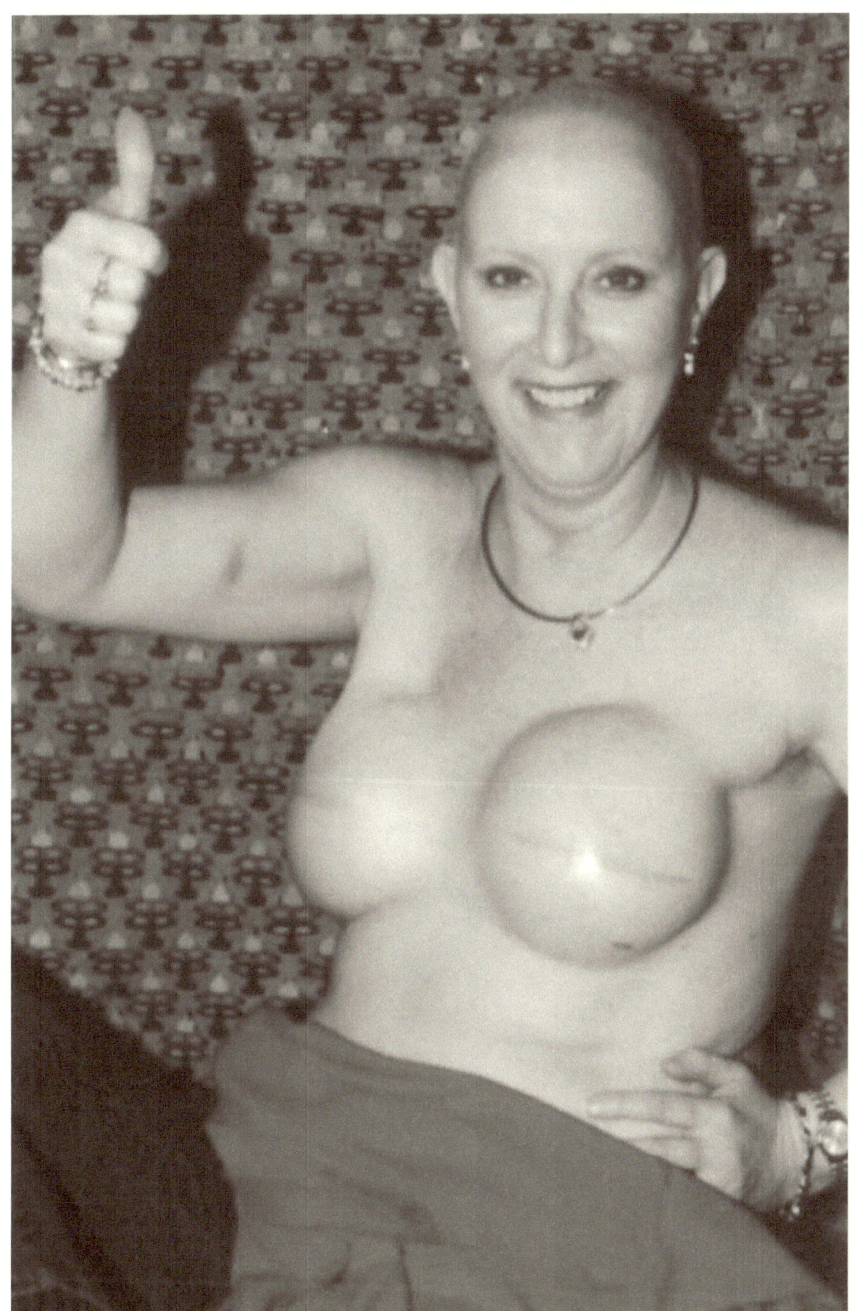

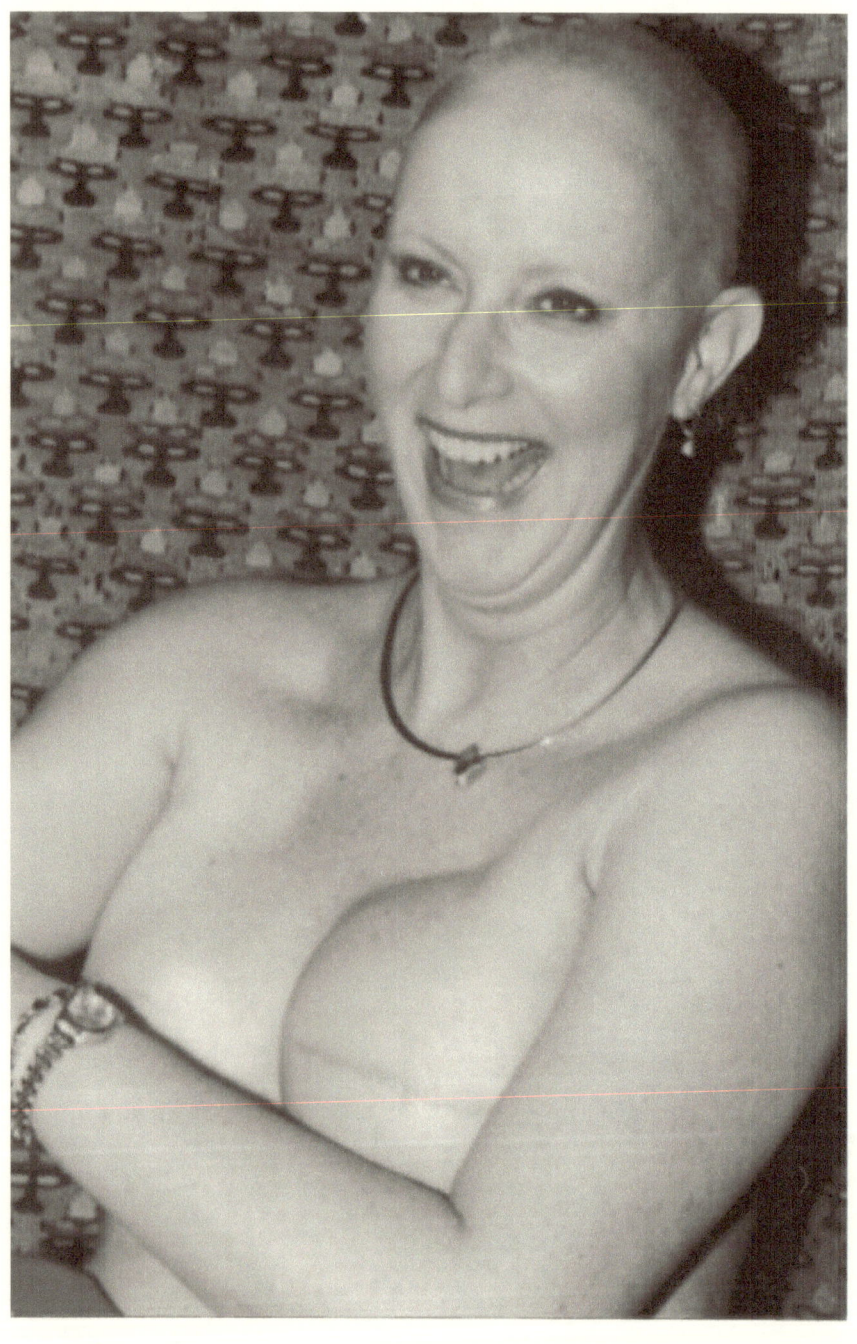

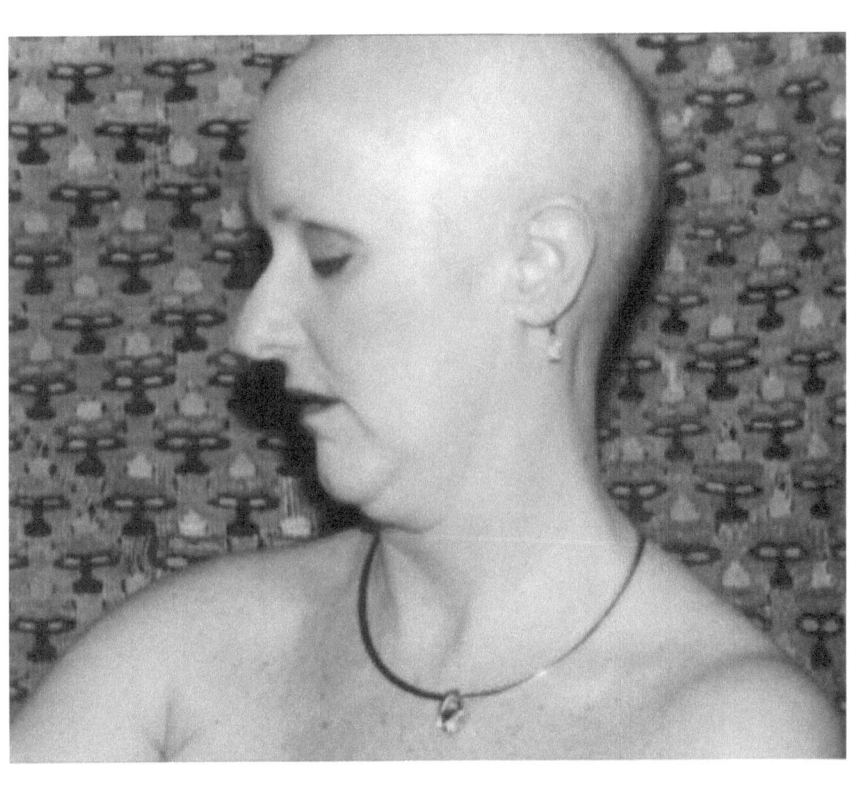

www.ingramcontent.com/pod-product-compliance
Lightning Source LLC
Chambersburg PA
CBHW050344290526
45785CB00006B/2631